CHRONIC LIVER DISEASES:

Understanding Liver Diseases

Eliane P. Barrera

Preface

Your liver is a giant and powerful organ that performs heaps of integral features in your body.
There are many kinds of liver disease. Some of the most frequent kinds are treatable with eating regimen and lifestyle changes, whilst others may additionally require lifelong remedy to manage.
Chronic liver ailment often won't cause symptoms in the early stages. But every so often it starts off evolving with an episode of acute hepatitis.
As liver disorder advances, it can affect your blood flow, hormones and dietary status. End-stage liver disorder refers to decompensated cirrhosis and liver failure, when your liver has misplaced the potential to regenerate and is slowly declining. Some sorts of liver illnesses have particular medical treatments. For example, antivirals treat viral hepatitis, while corticosteroids and immunosuppressants treat autoimmune diseases.

Contents

Introduction

There are many kinds of liver disease. Some of the most frequent kinds are treatable with eating regimen and lifestyle changes, whilst others may additionally require lifelong remedy to manage. If you commence remedy early enough, you can frequently stop permanent damage. But you can also now not have signs and symptoms in the early stages. Late-stage liver sickness is more complex to treat.

An overview of liver diseases

Your liver is a giant and powerful organ that performs heaps of integral features in your body. One of its most necessary features is filtering toxins from your blood. While your liver is well-equipped for this job, its function as a filter makes it susceptible to the toxins it processes. Too many toxins can crush your liver's assets and potential to function. This can occur temporarily or over a long duration of time.

When healthcare providers refer to liver disease, they're generally referring to chronic conditions that do modern harm to your liver over time. Viral infections, poisonous poisoning and sure metabolic conditions are amongst the common causes of chronic liver disease. Your liver has super regenerative powers, however continuously working additional time to restore itself takes its toll. Eventually, it can't keep up.

The ranges of chronic liver disease

Chronic liver disorder progresses in roughly four stages:

- Hepatitis.

- Fibrosis.

- Cirrhosis.

- Liver failure.

Stage 1: Hepatitis

Hepatitis ability irritation in your liver tissues. Inflammation is your liver's response to harm or toxicity. It's an attempt to purge infections and start the healing process. Acute hepatitis (an instantaneous and brief response) often accomplishes this. But when the harm or toxicity continues, so does the inflammation. Chronic hepatitis causes hyperactive recuperation that finally results in scarring (fibrosis).

Stage 2: Fibrosis

Fibrosis is a gradual stiffening of your liver as skinny bands of scar tissue progressively add up. Scar tissue reduces blood float through your liver, which reduces its admission to oxygen and nutrients. This is how your liver's vitality begins to regularly decline. Remarkably, some quantities of fibrosis are reversible. Your liver cells can regenerate, and scarring can scale back if the damage slows down enough for it to recover.

Stage 3: Cirrhosis

Cirrhosis is severe, everlasting scarring in your liver. This is the stage where fibrosis is no longer reversible. When your liver no longer has adequate healthy cells left to work with, its tissues can no longer regenerate. But you can still slow or quit the damage at this stage. Cirrhosis will start to have an effect on your liver function, but your physique will attempt to compensate for the loss, so you may now not notice at first.

Stage 4: Liver failure

Liver failure begins when your liver can no longer feature safely for your body's needs. This is also referred to as "decompensated cirrhosis" — your physique can no longer compensate for the losses. As liver features begin to wreck down, you'll begin to feel the effects throughout your body. Chronic liver failure is a gradual process, however it is eventually fatal barring a liver transplant. You want a liver to live.

Approximately 1.8% of U.S. adults (4.5 million adults) have liver disease. It reasons about 57,000 U.S. deaths a year. Globally, it reasons about 2 million deaths per year, or 4% of all deaths. Deaths are ordinarily from problems of cirrhosis, with acute liver failure accounting for a small portion. Liver disease affects guys and people assigned male at delivery (AMAB) twice as frequently as women and humans assigned girls at birth (AFAB).

Symptoms of liver diseases

The first signs and symptoms and signs of liver disease

Chronic liver ailment often won't cause symptoms in the early stages. But every so often it starts off evolving with an episode of acute hepatitis. For example, if you get a viral hepatitis infection, there's an acute section before the continual section sets in. You might have a fever, stomach ache or nausea for a quick duration while your immune system works to defeat the infection. If it doesn't defeat it, it will become a persistent infection.

Some different reasons for liver sickness could possibly also begin with more acute symptoms or have occasional episodes of acute symptoms. Early signs and symptoms of liver disease tend to be vague. They may include:

- Upper stomach pain.

- Nausea or loss of appetite.

- Fatigue and malaise (feeling generally worn-out and ill).

The signs and symptoms of later-stage liver disease

You would possibly start to note extra signs when your liver characteristic begins to decline. This happens in the later tiers of liver disease. One of the first facet results of declining liver feature is that bile glide stalls in your biliary tract. Your liver no longer produces or supplies bile correctly to your small intestine. Instead, bile starts off evolving to leak into your bloodstream. This motives unique symptoms, including:

- Jaundice (yellow tint to the whites of your eyes and skin).

- Dark-colored pee (urine).

- Light-colored poop (stool).

- Digestive difficulties, specifically with fats.

- Weight loss and muscle loss.

- Musty-smelling breath.

- Mild intelligence impairment (hepatic encephalopathy).

- Pruritus (itchy skin, however with no seen rash).

As liver disorder advances, it can affect your blood flow, hormones and dietary status. This can exhibit up in quite a number ways. You may additionally see signs and symptoms in your pores and skin and nails, such as:

- Spoon nails.

- Terry's nails.

- Nail clubbing.

- Spider angiomas.

- Tiny crimson dots on your skin (petechiae).

- Small yellow bumps of fats deposits on your skin or eyelids.

- Easy bleeding and bruising.

- Red fingers of your hands.

You may additionally see signs of fluids leaking from your blood vessels and amassing in your body, such as:

- Swollen abdomen (ascites).

- Swollen ankles, feet, palms and face (edema).

Liver sickness symptoms in humans assigned female at beginning may additionally include:

- Irregular periods (menstruation).

- Female infertility.

Liver sickness signs and symptoms in humans assigned male at beginning can also include:

- Shrunken testicles.

- Enlarged male breast tissue.

End-stage liver disorder refers to decompensated cirrhosis and liver failure, when your liver has misplaced the potential to regenerate and is slowly declining. The most huge side results of end-stage liver disease are portal hypertension and primary liver cancer (hepatocellular carcinoma). Complications of these two prerequisites are the main motives of hospitalization and loss of life in people with cirrhosis and liver failure.

Portal hypertension

Portal hypertension takes place when scarring in your liver compresses the portal vein that runs via it. High blood strain in the portal vein motives your physique to divert blood drift to other veins connected with it, which come to be enlarged and stretched thin. These veins can leak, wreck and bleed. Internal bleeding from these varices can be sudden, extreme and life-threatening.

Additional complications, although rare, include:

- Enlarged and overactive spleen (hypersplenism).

- Respiratory failure (hepatopulmonary syndrome).

- Kidney failure (hepatorenal syndrome).

Liver Cancer

While no longer absolutely everyone with chronic liver sickness gets major liver cancers (hepatocellular carcinoma), most people who do get liver cancer have persistent liver disease. The cycle of inflammation, repair and scarring changes your liver cells in approaches that make them greater likely to exchange into cancer. Healthcare providers also consider that chronic hepatitis viruses, in particular, might also intervene with the DNA in your liver cells.

There are over 100 types of liver disease, however they fall into a handful of subtypes. Causes include:

<u>Viral infections</u>

Viral hepatitis infections that come to be chronic can cause chronic hepatitis, including hepatitis A, hepatitis B and hepatitis C.

• Hepatitis A (Hep A) – This contamination is typically caused by consuming contaminated meals or water. This shape of hepatitis normally clears barring lasting problems within six months and does no longer lead to a continual infection. Typically, you can't get it extra than as soon as you consider the reasons for lifetime immunity after the first infection. A vaccine to prevent infection is available.

• Hepatitis B (Hep B) – This virus is transmitted through bodily fluids that triggers an immune reaction, causing low-level inflammation and liver damage. It is normally successfully dealt with with oral medications that have few side consequences or pegylated interferon injections. In a small number of cases, Hep B can develop into a persistent infection, which can lead to extra serious liver diseases. A vaccine to stop infection is available.

• Hepatitis C (Hep C) – Spread via contact with

infected blood, Hep C contamination can be very serious. Most people infected ride no signs and the virus may stay in the liver for years and it is no longer discovered until a lot of harm is done. It is an increasing number of successfully treated with pegylated interferon injections along with oral

drugs.

Up to 50 percent of those contaminated with Hepatitis C are able to fight off the virus within six months. However, many patients have a persistent infection. A liver biopsy can determine the extent of harm and harm to the liver.

Treatment includes antiviral medicines, such as pegylated interferon and ribavirin, to limit liver damage.

<u>Alcohol-induced hepatitis.</u>

Heavy alcohol use can cause acute or continual hepatitis. If it goes on long enough, it can cause cirrhosis and liver failure.

Toxic hepatitis

Chronic overexposure to toxins, such as industrial chemical substances or drugs, can cause acute or continual hepatitis.

Non-alcohol related fatty liver disease

Metabolic conditions associated with obesity, high blood sugar and excessive blood lipids can cause extra fat storage in your liver, which can cause infection (non-alcohol related steatohepatitis).

Biliary stasis

Congenital (present at birth) stipulations that hinder or stall the waft of bile via your bile ducts can cause bile to construct up and injure your liver, including biliary atresia and cystic fibrosis. Non-congenital reasons include biliary stricture and gallstones.

Autoimmune liver diseases

Autoimmune conditions can motivate continued inflammation and scarring in your liver or your bile ducts, including autoimmune hepatitis, primary biliary cholangitis and primary sclerosing cholangitis.

. Primary sclerosing cholangitis (PSC) – This disease causes the liver's bile ducts to turn out to be inflamed, scarred and finally blocked. This can lead to cholangitis, a condition of bacterial contamination of the bile, and cirrhosis.

Treatment includes medicine to relieve itching, antibiotics, anti-inflammatories, bile thinners and diet supplements. PSC is often related with inflammatory bowel disease (IBD), which may additionally require cure on its own.

PSC can cause liver failure and additionally is a dangerous thing for developing bile duct cancer, for that reason shut followup is required.

• Primary biliary cirrhosis (PBC) – PBC is some other disease

that destroys the liver's bile ducts, causing bile to accumulate in the liver and injure liver tissue. Initial treatment is usually aimed at providing symptom relief and includes vitamin therapy, calcium dietary supplements and tablets to treat itching. Bile thinners and anti-infl ammatory medications are also usually used. While the sickness can't be cured, its progression can also be delayed. However, if the liver turns into severely damaged, a transplant may additionally be necessary.

• Autoimmune hepatitis – This is a condition in which the body assaults the liver, causing the liver to become inflamed and scarred (hepatitis). If identified and treated early, autoimmune hepatitis can typically be effectively controlled.

Treatment typically consists of a aggregate of medications and corticosteroids to gradual down the overactive immune gadgets and stop the ailments from getting worse, and perhaps reverse some of the damage.

<u>Inherited metabolic disorders</u>

Disorders that cause toxic merchandise to build up in your blood — such as glycogen storage disease (GSD), Wilson disease, hemochromatosis and Gaucher disease — can motivate persistent liver damage.

• Hereditary Hemochromatosis – The most common adult genetic liver ailment in which a specific genetic defect leads to iron accumulation in the liver, leading to liver cirrhosis and liver most cancers in some patients. Iron accumulation may also go beyond the liver affecting the heart,

joints and pancreas. Specific and high-quality treatments are available. Liver transplantation may additionally be required in some of these patients.

• Alpha-1 antitrypsin deficiency (Alpha-1) – This inherited disease may additionally have an effect on the liver and/or the lungs in children and adults. It is caused via an inability to produce enough

of a particular protein, called Alpha-1 antitrypsin, which is used to forestall the breakdown of enzymes in various organs. Management of Alpha-1 antitrypsin deficiency includes patient education, retaining regular nutrition, and carefully monitoring patients so that any complications

can be handled early. There are potential scientific trials for medical therapies. Liver transplantation efficaciously cures the condition.

• Wilson's sickness – A uncommon genetic ailment that reasons excessive buildup of copper in the liver and brain.

Treatment is managed by way of each hepatologist and neurologist and includes oral medication, which binds to the copper and removes it from the body. Therapy is endured to prevent its reaccumulation.

• Hereditary amyloidosis – A circumstance in which the liver produces an atypical protein that builds up in other organs, causing problems in the nerves and kidneys. Treatment consists of medicinal drugs or different healing procedures to avoid protein buildup, or a liver transplant to quit disease progression and prevent similar harm to other organs.

<u>Cardiovascular diseases</u>

Conditions that have an effect on blood waft to and from your liver — including Budd-Chiari syndrome, ischemia, arterial illnesses and right-sided coronary heart failure — can purpose continual liver damage.

Hazard factors for obtaining liver disease

You may also be greater probable to get liver ailment if you:

- Drink alcohol heavily.

- Use intravenous drugs.

- Use pain relievers like aspirin or acetaminophen

- Have metabolic syndrome.

- Are regularly uncovered to toxic chemicals.

- Are often exposed to different people's blood or physique fluids.

Diagnosis and Tests

Test for liver disease

A healthcare provider checking for liver ailment will begin through physically examining you. They'll appear for visible symptoms and ask about your symptoms. They may also ask about your diet, life-style and fitness history. Finally, they'll use lab tests and imaging scans to test for liver disease. These might also include:

Blood tests

A panel of liver feature tests can show symptoms of liver disease, liver disorder severity and liver failure. These measure liver merchandise like liver enzymes, proteins and bilirubin levels in your blood. Blood exams may additionally point out inflammation, specific illnesses or facet effects, like decreased blood clotting.

Imaging tests

An abdominal ultrasound, CT scan (computed tomography scan) or MRI (magnetic resonance imaging) can exhibit the size, structure and texture of your liver. This can expose infection and swelling, growths and fibrosis.

Elastography.

A distinctive type of imaging check known elastography uses ultrasound or MRI technology to measure the level of stiffness or fibrosis in your liver.

Endoscopy

If your provider wants to see the inside of your biliary tract, they may need to use a type of endoscopic imaging. Endoscopy entails passing a tiny digicam (endoscope) through your higher GI tract. From the endoscope, they can use EUS or ERCP to see your bile ducts.

Nuclear medicinal drug imaging

A nuclear liver and spleen scan uses a gamma digicam to observe a (harmless) radioactive tracer material that's injected into your body. How your liver absorbs the tracer will highlight the areas that aren't functioning normally.

Liver biopsy

A liver biopsy is a minor system to take a small tissue pattern from your liver to take a look at in a lab. A healthcare provider can generally take the sample through a hole needle. You would possibly need a liver biopsy to test for most cancers or confirm cirrhosis and help decide the cause.

How to treat liver disease

Some sorts of liver illnesses have particular medical treatments. For example, antivirals treat viral hepatitis, while corticosteroids and immunosuppressants treat autoimmune diseases. But in many cases, lifestyle modifications are the major treatment for liver disease. Reducing the poisonous load on your liver is vital with any kind of liver disease, however integral for those brought on via extra fats storage, alcohol or different toxins.

However, early recognition is key to treating liver disorder effectively earlier than everlasting damage is done. Unfortunately, no longer absolutely everyone discovers liver sickness in time to reverse its course. If you already have cirrhosis or liver failure, you would possibly want additional redress for complications like portal hypertension or liver cancer. Your liver may now not be able to recover, and you might finally want a liver transplant.

Ways you can decrease danger of liver disease

You can assist prevent liver disease by:

Getting vaccinated. Vaccines are reachable to stop viral hepatitis A and B.

Practice suitable hygiene. Handwashing after using the bathroom, protected meals managing and safe needle use can assist stop infections from spreading.

Drinking alcohol in moderation and the usage of medicines as directed. If you have a substance use disorder (SUD), treatment can help prevent poisonous hepatitis.

Managing metabolic factors such as your blood lipids and blood sugar. A healthcare issuer can assist with this.

Can liver sickness be reversed?

Liver disorder can be reversed in the early ranges if you and your healthcare group are capable of eliminating or controlling the motive effectively. This depends on the motive and how treatable it is. Once you have cirrhosis, you can't undo the scarring that's already been done, however you can also be able to prevent in addition damage or gradual it down. Chronic liver failure isn't reversible, though it can nevertheless take years to progress.

Is liver ailment curable?

Many types of liver ailment are curable. Toxic and alcohol-related liver disease can improve when you're no longer exposed to the toxin. Diet and lifestyle changes can relieve non-alcohol related fatty liver disease. Other types of liver disease aren't curable, but they're often manageable with medications. Certain inherited diseases, autoimmune diseases and viral infections may additionally want lifelong treatment.

Ways you can take care of yourself while residing with liver disease

If you have liver disease, you can help take care of your liver by:

Maintaining a healthful diet. Emphasize whole foods, with plenty of plants and lean protein.

Maintaining a healthy BMI (body mass index). Your healthcare issuer can advise you.

Avoiding alcohol, tobacco and nonprescription drug use. Ask your healthcare provider for resources to help you quit.

Taking medicinal drugs solely as directed. Always talk about any new medicinal drugs with your provider.

Protecting yourself from infections. Practice appropriate hygiene and secure intercourse to avoid additional burdens on your liver.

Keeping up with your healthcare appointments. Get your regular screenings to capture complications early.